Me, Myself & Food

Conquering The Struggle Against
Overweight & Obesity
Without Dieting

To Chris -
All the best in
health & life!

Tiara Hunter

Me, Myself & Food
Conquering The Struggle Against Overweight & Obesity Without Dieting

by Diana Hunter

Consumer Press
Fort Lauderdale

Published by:
Consumer Press
13326 Southwest 28th Street, Suite 102
Fort Lauderdale, FL 33330-1102

The author, publisher, and any and all affiliated parties with regard to the production of this book shall have neither liability nor responsibility to any person, property, entity, or organization whatsoever with respect to any loss or damage whatsoever caused, or alleged to be caused, directly or indirectly, by the information contained herein. This book is sold with the understanding that the publisher is not engaged in rendering nutritional, medical, or other professional service. If medical advice or other expert assistance is required, the services of an appropriate professional should be sought. Although all efforts have been made to ensure correctness, the author and publisher assume no responsibility for errors, omissions, or inaccuracies.

Common sense is a virtue. If you are clinically obese, have any other form of health problem, are on medication of any kind, have a family history of any type of disease, or are pregnant or attempting to become pregnant, be sure to consult fully with one or more qualified medical professionals before making nutrition-related lifestyle changes. Good health is a team effort that begins with, and is directed by, you. Even if you believe yourself to be in good or relatively good health, having a qualified medical professional monitor your progress can be an asset. In addition, due to the ever-changing and debatable nature of nutrition, information contained in this book may not reflect every up-to-the-minute perspective.

Library of Congress Cataloging in Publication Data
Hunter, Diana, 1961-
Me, myself & food : conquering the struggle against overweight and obesity without dieting / by Diana Hunter.
pages cm
Includes bibliographic references and index.
ISBN-13: 978-1-891264-68-9 (pbk. : alk. paper)
ISBN-10: 1-891264-68-0 (pbk. : alk. paper)
1. Weight loss--Psychological aspects. 2. Obesity--Psychological aspects. 3. Self-care, Health. I. Title. II. Title: Me, myself and food.
RM222.2.H8597 2012
613.2'5--dc23
2012036022

ISBN-13: 978-1-891264-68-9 / ISBN-10: 1-891264-68-0 $12.95 Softcover

10 9 8 7 6 5 4 3 2
Printed in the United States of America

Table of Contents

About The Author

Diana Hunter is an award-winning author, nutrition researcher, and college instructor who holds a degree in food science. Her background includes certification in food safety and management as well as studies and awards in the behavioral sciences.

Her previous literary achievements include *FoodSmart: Understanding Nutrition in the 21st Century* and *The Ritalin-Free Child: Managing Hyperactivity & Attention Deficits Without Drugs*, a Parents' Choice Approval Award winner. She has been seen and heard on hundreds of network stations throughout the country as part of her acclaimed "Be FoodSmart" National Tour, and has presented at numerous colleges, universities, bookstores, libraries, and nutrition-related venues. Founder of the FoodSmart Alliance, she is also the developer of FoodSmart Nutrition, a course currently offered at various colleges, and is a recent recipient of a Broward College Hall of Distinction Award.

Ms. Hunter's goal is to help educate others about nutrition and health on a global scale, with a focus on helping those with weight issues and debilitating illnesses. She is a firm believer in the idea that *health* reform, rather than *healthcare* reform, will lead to a healthier society, and that preventive care is the key to achieving it.

She resides in Fort Lauderdale, Florida.

For every person who has ever struggled with weight issues and wished for a better way.

In loving memory of
Elaine Gibertini,
who helped keep the candle burning.

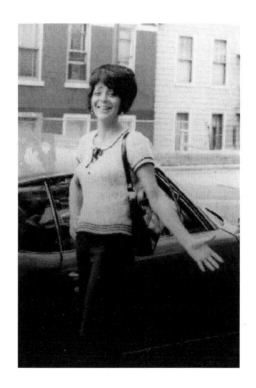

Acknowledgements

Special thanks to my family (Steve, Tony, and Brenden), Cici Petersen, Gerda Williams, Rita Ion, Kimba Nichols, Winona Golden, Joseph Pappas, Diane Lentini, Vito Lentini, Linda Muzzarelli, Gina Muzzarelli, Jesse Ruggles, Rebekah Ruggles, Shawna Thompson, Dan Poynter, and the late Jan Nathan.

Special thanks is also extended to the many researchers, reviewers, and others around the globe who have provided assistance and permissions during the development of this book and its related projects, as well as to Salvatore Concialdi of Concialdi Design for his artistry, intuition, and patience and the staff of Southern WebWorks for their continued and exceptional service, solutions, support, and attention to detail at a moment's notice. Your efforts are appreciated!

Introduction

If you've tried every diet-related pill, plan, and powder and weigh more than when you started, or you simply can't get a grip on weight loss or weight maintenance, take heart. You're by no means a failure. You've simply been missing a vital tool. It's called self-perspective. And you need to know how to use it effectively.

This book has been designed to help you see the real obstacles that keep you from losing weight or maintaining a healthy weight and how to move beyond them so you can achieve a slim, healthy you for life. It has nothing to do with being on a diet. In fact, it's the ultimate anti-diet book. It's an anti-diet book with a built-in road map for success.

The truth is, when it comes to basic, there's-no-health-emergency weight loss, you don't need to be on a diet. Ever. You just need to learn how to eat right and use your self-perspective to your greatest advantage. My goal within these pages is to help you accomplish just that.

As you journey through this book, you'll gain new insight into your personal relationship—or lack thereof—with food, and be able to develop a promising new outlook on nutrition-related self-care.

Combining a new viewpoint on how you see yourself with regard to food, and vice-versa, is easy once you know how, and can effectively and successfully lead to conquering your weight issues for life. Just set your sights on it and put your mind to it. You're worth it. You deserve it. You *can* do it!

Diana Hunter
November 2012

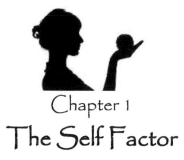

Chapter 1

The Self Factor

elieve it or not, how you see yourself plays an important role in your ability to lose or maintain weight. In fact, it pretty much dictates how successful you can be at either one. Mind you, I'm not talking about how you see yourself in terms of *what* you see when you look in the mirror. I'm talking about *who* you see. You know, it's that self-love thing you've heard about—or are even tired of hearing about. But before you close the book, let me assure you that my goal here isn't to get you to dig deep into your psyche to find out if you love yourself or not. Rather, it's to provide you with a factual overview of the things that affect your weight so you can take control of them once and for all and live your life free from dieting. They include genuinely caring about yourself. Simply stated, self-love is at the forefront of everything in your life, including your food choices and your food intake, and to make any real, lasting change you have to lasso it. It's what allows you to control your eating, rather than allowing your eating to control you.

Don't be fooled, however. Being overweight or obese isn't solely a psychological issue. It's both a psychological and physical one. It's also an academic one, because having at least a basic understanding of how the body works and how different foods and nutrients affect it are essential pieces of the puzzle. Still, your overall mental outlook and perspectives, particularly about yourself, play the top roles that influence your food-related actions, for better or worse. The bottom line is that if you're willing to work on improving yourself, both the time and effort you put in will pay off in some really big ways.

So how does one begin to effectively navigate the ocean of self-love as quickly and easily as possible? By taking a (very) brief tour of the Big Five: Self-Respect, Self-Care, Self-Esteem, Health, and Determination. Each of these interlocks with the others. Together, they equal success. Your success. For life.

#1 Self-Respect. Self-respect means protecting your body—physically, mentally, or otherwise—from negative influences, including those you can inflict upon yourself (read: poor diet habits). It's easy to achieve self-respect if you already love, or at least like, yourself. But if you don't, no worries. You can start right now. Just consider the incredible machine your body is. If you're healthy and fortunate, you can think, hear, see, taste, touch, smell, and much more. Now consider waking up tomorrow morning without one or more of those options, or with less options than you currently have. Not too appealing. Could make a bad day/situation/life worse. So start appreciating what you have (even if you're ill), remind yourself that you're worth it as often as necessary (even if you think you're not), and start protecting your body (even if you don't really feel like it). In the same way that the simple act of smiling can make you feel happier, these actions alone will promote you to care about yourself. If you feel you need help, professional or otherwise, to heal emotional wounds or overcome addictions that might deter your efforts, get it. There are also plenty of good self-help resources, including books, if that's more your style. Or you can just take my word for it that you're worth it and go from there. Every day is a new opportunity to start over and take better care of yourself. Seize them all.

#2 Self-Care. Self-care encompasses all the positive, healthful things you do for yourself—physically, mentally, or otherwise—including those related to food and nutrition. If you respect yourself and are determined to take care of yourself, you'll have an easier time making strides toward weight loss and weight maintenance and you'll achieve better health. This will likely mean completely overhauling your diet. It will definitely mean reading labels (and learning *how* to read them), avoiding most chemical ingredients, and finding alternatives to certain foods (see chapter 4 for alternative food suggestions). You may also have to start eating differently from others, including your family members. Familial eating patterns, not "overweight genes from my parents" are often "inherited" from previous generations and can have catastrophic consequences, including childhood obesity and self-induced diabetes. There are solutions, however. Years ago, after realizing he didn't want to be overweight and ill, my teenage nephew separated both his fridge and pantry at home into two sections—his and the rest of the family's. His sections included whole grain foods and foods that were low in sodium, sugar, fat, and chemical additives. The effect was amazing, and he's never gone back to his old eating habits. You can do it too. Remember, you're worth it. And don't get lazy about it. Once you start practicing self-care, the rest will follow.

#3 Self-Esteem. Self-esteem is one of the gifts you automatically receive when you practice self-respect and self-care. Food is no longer controlling you. You are controlling it. You decide what to eat, how to prepare it, and how much of it to eat. You look and feel better, and can take pride in your accomplishments. Recognize and enjoy your boost in confidence and use it to keep promoting your efforts.

#4 Health. Better health is another gift you automatically receive when you change your eating habits.

You will very likely feel better, have less pain, spend less on doctor visits and medications, and enjoy a higher quality of life. For *years*. And just think of the financial benefits, not only for you, but everyone else too. You can take pride in the fact that you are being personally responsible for your health and doing your part to help lessen healthcare costs. One person *can* make a difference. Start learning more about health, particularly from a nutritional perspective (see chapter 4 for help in this area), and you'll benefit even more. It takes some work, but again, you're worth it. Be diligent. You can do it.

#5 Determination. Being determined means not giving up, no matter what. If you're determined to respect your body, you will. And you'll lose weight and feel better. It's a win-win situation from a lot of different angles. You're in control of your own fork. You have the power to make changes. Just stay focused. Never quit.

Making It Happen

Now that you know what it takes to make progress toward your weight-related goals, the next step is to actually start applying what you know. Not just thinking about it, but *doing* it. If, for example, you use food as a crutch during stressful times, do a little research to find tasty, healthier alternative foods to munch on when you're stressed. (I can hear you groaning about testing different foods and the cost to do so, but it'll be worth it. It's a lot less expensive than medical bills and missed work days.) Don't forget about basic, unprocessed foods like fruits and vegetables. Then work on finding a healthy alternative outlet for your stress. You may be shocked to find that in a lot of instances you'll actually be able to eat *more* than you ate before without gaining weight. You may also be surprised to find that your desire for junk foods and foods high in fat, sodium, and sugar will decline and your appetite for an overall healthier lifestyle will increase.

One bit of advice: if you're thinking about taking what you think will be a shortcut, don't. Not unless you absolutely have to. By this I mean don't have gastric bypass surgery or any other type of surgical weight loss procedure unless your doctor says it's absolutely necessary. Why? **Because you're still going to have to learn how to eat right.** Once you have the surgery you'll be told what you can and can't (or should I say should or shouldn't) eat. And beware: if you don't follow the rules, the consequences can be, well, awful. Cheat a little and the food may go right through you. God forbid in public. Or, if you're like one of my old friends from college, you may experience a life-threatening side effect from the surgery and nearly die. Given these considerations, along with the costs and downtime associated with surgery, just plain learning to eat right starts to sound pretty good to most people. Some even step it up a notch and buy a home gym or start going to spin class.

A Beneficial Perspective

Overall, getting to know yourself from a physical and nutritional standpoint is important if for no other reason than the fact that your dietary needs are unique. For instance, while some people have an issue with eating before going to sleep, it's almost essential for others. I usually eat a large bowl of high-fiber, low-sugar cereal with organic, low-fat, lactose-free milk right before I go to bed. I sleep exceptionally well and my digestive tract is quite happy with the arrangement. You may or may not find that the same thing works for you. Generally speaking, your individual nutritional requirements and situations are most likely very different from mine, your neighbor's, your partner's, and even those of your parents and siblings. Nutrition is not "one size fits all." Understanding your own nutritional profile is an important facet of the self factor that will empower you to control your weight for life.

Motives For Motivation

Considering your weight-loss motives is also important. One reason the self-love aspect is so essential in your quest to lose weight is that when you try to lose it solely to impress others it's usually a short-lived effort. When you do it for yourself, however, the effort becomes virtually effortless—and often has lasting effects. However, keep in mind that there are instances in which when you lose weight to *benefit* others, rather than to *impress* them, it's a totally different scenario. In these cases you still benefit yourself first and foremost. They just benefit at the same time. I call it The Oxygen Mask Theory. Consider those little oxygen masks in airplanes that drop down when cabin pressure drops. The flight attendant always tells you to put yours on first before assisting others. Same concept with weight loss. The healthier you are, the better you can take care of your family, pets, and so on. And just think of the example you set for others. You're not only in control, but you're also sharing the gift of good health. Priceless.

Beating The Odds

During your weight-loss or weight-maintenance journey you may run into hurdles. Don't panic. You can jump, remove, or at least manage all of them. That is, if you really want to. Determination needs to become, and remain, your new best friend. That doesn't mean you can never eat your favorite junk food (unless that's your choice). It also doesn't mean you need to walk around hungry, or eat foods that are flavorless or taste bad. It does, however, mean that if you falter you'll get right back up and keep going. It means you'll give it your best effort and you won't give up, no matter what. It means you'll be persistent against all odds. It means you'll build a new relationship with food. Just remember to stay focused on the overall outcome—in other words, on all the benefits of getting to and staying at a healthy weight.

Use the self factor to your advantage. Knowing about yourself will help you keep from getting in your own way.

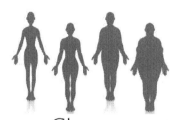

Chapter 2
Overweight:
Prelude To Obesity

Pounds are sneaky. They creep up on you while you're working, going to college, raising your family, or remodeling the house. In other words, while you're busy living your life. You repeatedly resign yourself to the idea that you'll start a diet on Monday, but you always:

a) have to eat the leftovers so they don't go to waste,

b) have someone offer to cook you homemade lasagna or some other specialty you can't resist,

c) get taken on a date to a five-star restaurant,

d) encounter a 2-for-1 sale on your favorite ice cream,

e) get invited to a party/baby shower/employee luncheon where the food is simply amazing,

f) realize a holiday is right around the corner and put off dieting until after it passes, or

g) have some other reason.

Or you start a diet and *then* one of these things happens. Worse yet, you play the blame game. Some examples: the boss keeps bringing in donuts and bagels and you're forced to eat them to show your appreciation (or to suck up); you travel a lot for work and the only convenient foods you can get your hands on are in vending machines and are high in fat, sodium, sugar, and chemical additives (or some combination of these); your spouse or significant other "forces" you to eat a big meal every night at 8:30 p.m. when he or she gets home. You get the picture. These are excuses for weight gain, not reasons.

The fact is, dieting takes effort. It's work. So is learning to eat right. But in the race between the two, learning to feed yourself in a way that benefits you as an individual will win hands down every time. And you only have to learn how to eat right *once*. After that the template for knowing what to buy and eat stays pretty much the same. You just can't beat it.

A Double-Edged Sword

One thing it's important not to lose sight of is the fact that extra weight affects far more than your looks. "It's not a death sentence," you may think. Think again. Deaths related to obesity claim somewhere in the vicinity of 112,000 lives every year according to the CDC. And overweight leads to obesity. Health conditions and illnesses associated with both overweight and obesity include:

- Type 2 diabetes
- Hypertension (High blood pressure)
- Heart disease
- Stroke
- Arthritis
- Breast cancer
- Reproductive problems
- Digestive difficulties
- Colon cancer
- Gallbladder disease
- Fatty liver
- Breathing problems
- Physical disabilities
- Erectile dysfunction
- Sleep difficulties
- Thyroid problems

That's a lot of illnesses, and they're affecting a lot of people. The CDC's 2010 report on overweight and obesity statistics in the U.S. shows that between 2007 and 2008 alone 34% of adults 20 years of age and older were overweight. Another 34% were reported as being obese. That's 68% of the adult population. And that just may be a low estimate.

Unfortunately, kids aren't faring much better. In fact, their odds are worse simply because they're kids. The fact that they may have more time on their hands now may also mean they have less time later in terms of life expectancy. The childhood statistics for 2007 to 2008 showed that 10% of kids age 2-5, 20% of kids age 6-11, and 18% of kids age 12-19 were obese.

As with anything else, knowing the cause is the key to prevention—or elimination—of the problem. Here are just some of the causes (and potential causes) of overweight, as well as situations that can lead to it:

- Poor diet and eating habits (childhood included)
- Overeating as a result of food addictions
- Lack of exercise or physical activity
- Sedentary lifestyles (office workers, work-at-home typists, and others who don't exercise regularly)
- Pregnancy
- Post-childbirth issues
- Perimenopause
- Menopause
- Postmenopause
- Diabetes, overactive thyroid, or other illness
- Stress, anxiety, and/or depression
- Serious injury
- Handicaps
- Age
- Location

- Poor sleep habits or inability to sleep
- Medications
- Quitting smoking
- Water retention
- Joint problems
- Headaches & migraines

Note that hormonal imbalances are not on this list. That's because, even though you often hear of them being referred to as a reason for weight gain, they are *extremely* rare in and of themselves. There's virtually always a detectable reason when our hormones are out of whack. For example, while a malfunctioning thyroid may produce less thyroid hormone and you may subsequently gain weight, it is in effect your thyroid issues, and not your hormones, that started the trouble.

In other cases hormones are just innocent bystanders. The hormone changes that take place during perimenopause, for example, do not cause weight gain. Rather, perimenopause is *correlated* with weight gain, meaning women tend to gain weight during this time period. What's really ironic in the whole "hormones are making me fat" thing is the fact that obesity itself is actually a *cause* of hormonal imbalance.

The Metabolism Myth

Another misconception a lot of people have is that their metabolism causes them to gain weight. People often tell me that theirs is "ultra-slow or "barely functioning." If in fact this were true, it would mean they were on the brink of death. True disruptive changes in metabolism that can cause weight gain are most often caused by serious medical conditions such as hypothyroidism, or by medications—and they're *very* rare.

Your Basal Metabolic Rate, or BMR, which is the rate at which your body burns calories just to keep you alive (it's generally calculated as the amount we burn while we sleep) is what most people refer to as their metabolism. But it's only one factor in calorie burning—and it's a pretty stable one. The most important factor is physical activity (read: good old-fashioned exercise). The goal is to use up at least as many calories as we take in. To lose weight, we have to burn even more calories, take in less calories, or both. To boot, while your BMR does have a genetic link, and you could come close to or even match your grandmother's baseline BMR during her older years (BMR declines as you age), you can actually *increase* your BMR with exercise, sleep, water, and healthy food. Imagine that.

The Difference Between Overweight & Obesity

So at what point does overweight end and obesity begin? The most common tool used to figure it out is the body mass index, or BMI, a number that shows body weight adjusted for height. For most adults, a BMI of:

- under 18.5 indicates underweight

- 18.5 to 24.9 indicates normal weight

- 25 to 29.9 indicates overweight

- 30 or over indicates obesity

While the BMI generally provides a quick estimate of a person's body fat, it's not always accurate. This is because it doesn't measure body fat directly. Therefore, those who have enhanced muscle mass, such as athletes, body builders, and construction workers, may have misleading BMI results. Their muscle mass adds weight, just like fat does, though it's unlikely to cause the same health problems. However, it's important to keep in mind that excess weight of any type may damage the body's joints, among other things. A BMI of 30 or more is usually a good indicator that an adult has too much body fat—a risky scenario that leaves one exposed to a host of health problems.

For both children and adolescents, the word "overweight" is used instead of "obese" for a BMI that is at or above the 95 percentile for a specific sex and age.

To quickly calculate your BMI online, go to **www.cdc.gov/nccdphp/dnpa/bmi/index.htm** and use the handy BMI calculator they provide. Or you can calculate it yourself using the following formula:

$$\text{weight (lbs)} / [\text{height (in)}]^2 \times 703$$

Divide weight (lbs) by height (in) squared, and then multiply by a conversion factor of 703.

Example: Weight = 150 lbs, Height = 5'5" (65")
Calculation: $[150 \div (65)^2] \times 703 = 24.96$

For those who are healthy, fending off weight shouldn't be that much of a problem. While there are some exceptions (most of which are correctable medical problems), recall that there is one simple equation that works for virtually everyone: when the amount of calories we take in and the amount of calories we burn is equivalent, our weight stays basically the same. What's really important is the *type* of calories we take in. For example, it's healthier to eat a given amount of carbs in the form of a bowl of oat bran than to eat the same amount of carbs in a couple of slices of toast made from bleached white flour. That's whole carbs versus refined carbs. Your body knows the difference. I know this firsthand from personal experience—and a whole lot of research. At the age of twenty-one, after passing out repeatedly for days, I was clinically diagnosed as hypoglycemic. I was also found to have allergies to a few different foods, including cane sugar, almonds, raisins, and peanuts. Working sixteen-hour days and eating trail mix that contained all those ingredients about every six hours or so explained my constant fainting spells. Throw in some cigarettes and several cups of coffee every day and the outcome wasn't good. I met with a dietician, who put me on a diet of fruit, vegetables, and meat—and included applesauce and cin-namon-sugared graham crackers. When I asked why she wanted me to eat the sugared graham crackers she said, "Well you have to have some fun food!" I tried it her way for a while. I had no relief. That's when I disregarded the new diet plan she gave me and focused on whole grains, vegetables, nuts and seeds I wasn't allergic to, lean meat, boiled eggs, and whole fruit eaten with low-fat organic cheese. What a difference. I've never turned back.

Learning about my food allergies and the fact that I had low blood sugar made me sort of an accidental tourist in the world of nutrition. In a good way. I chose to eat eggs because they were fast, easy, and full of protein. I'd run out the door every second or third morning with one boiled egg and a piece of real whole grain toast (read: read the labels for ingredients and fiber content). And I felt great after I ate them. On the other mornings I would eat a bowl of hot oat bran or whole grain cereal with low-fat organic milk. I'd also snack on a small amount of raw walnuts or other nuts throughout the day, but instead of eating them every six hours or so I'd eat them every couple of hours. I still eat this way today. I'm now fifty, and being overweight has never been an issue.

As a side note, people often question why I don't eat egg whites rather than whole eggs. The way I see it, there are no design errors in eggs. So why should I take them apart? Besides, not only do they contain every vitamin except vitamin C, but they also have some amazing benefits, especially for our eyes and livers, in the *yolk*. Plus, I eat a diet rich in cholesterol-taming food, including my oat bran, and **food isn't the only thing that raises cholesterol levels**. Eggs in moderation—or minimization—(about two to three a week) can actually help you keep your weight down. (Be sure to check with your doctor first if you have cholesterol issues or are on cholesterol-reducing medication before making any egg-related diet changes.) Just keep in mind that when prepared scrambled or as an omelet, most restaurants' idea of "one" egg is more like three or four...or five. And then there's the butter or oil they cook them in to consider.

The sugar allergy thing seemed crazy to me at first. How could I possibly avoid sugar? It was in almost everything. (Now it's been mostly replaced by corn syrup in products, which, contrary to what that commercial says about the body recognizing it "the same as sugar" is certainly not true for me, as I'm not allergic to corn.) So soda, candy, pastries, and a lot of other stuff sort of became off limits unless I made it myself without the cane sugar or ran into a really crafty baker. I swapped out any type of sugary drink for seltzer water or plain water, adding only a little lemon or fruit juice for flavor. Little did I know at the time that I was setting my body up to be a lean machine for life.

Along the way I learned an effective tactic for stopping weight gain and reversing it. It's to use what I call "The Quota System." I use it to control the amount of sugar I consume, cane or otherwise. It's how I regulate eating "fun" food. For example, if I want to have a small piece of pastry that contains added sugar, I'll avoid all other added-sugar foods that day. I save my added-sugar "quota" for the treat. This same quota system can be used for fat, carb, sodium, protein, and natural sugar (like in fruit) intake too. It's easy to do once you get used to which foods are best for you. And it's a lot easier than counting calories will ever be.

If you mess up, no problem. You can pay yourself back on The Quota System. Just skip any sugary, high-fat, or high-sodium foods the next day and do some form of moderate exercise for an extra hour. All you have to do is keep a mental (or written) tab of what you owe yourself. Let your conscience be your guide. It has one hell of a memory. By the way, with all the paybacks you pay back, you gain muscle tone. Nice.

All in all, it's essential to keep an eye on your eating habits. It's particularly important to watch your intake of saturated fat, and to altogether eliminate your consumption of trans fat because it reduces your HDL, or "good" cholesterol. However, you shouldn't attempt to cut *all* saturated fat out of your diet. Why? Because it's found in beneficial plant-based foods such as olive oil in addition to animal-based foods such as meat and milk. Your body needs good fats to function.

You also need to keep moving, especially as you get older (see chapter 8 for information on exercise). If you're eating properly and exercising regularly and you start gaining weight unexplainably, see your doctor.

The overall message: tackle your weight before it tackles you.

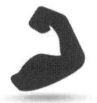

Chapter 3
Willpower:
A Better Way To Use It

C onquering overweight and obesity is a lot easier than you think. Contrary to popular belief, it doesn't require strict diets, costly eating plans, massive food restrictions, or sixty hours of diehard exercise a week. What it does require, once you've got the self-love thing down pat, is the knowledge of how to use your willpower effectively. And it's most likely not the way you think.

Rather than using your willpower to keep yourself from buying and eating certain foods and beverages—in other words, living in a constant state of restriction—you need to use it to focus on learning about different types of foods, how they can benefit or harm your health, and what your potential alternatives are. A case scenario: You walk into a grocery store and a clerk is placing freshly made fruit pies on a display table. They're still warm. The aroma is simply amazing. Blueberries are your favorite food...and the blueberry one looks the best. It's your move. What are you going to do? Here are three potential outcomes:

1) You approach the pie table. You can't resist the temptation. The look, the aroma...the dollar off! The pie is officially adopted. It's tucked carefully into your shopping cart along with your other "selections." You take it home and end up eating most (or all) of it yourself. Next.

2) You completely avoid the pie table. Later you pig out on a different dessert-type food. The next time you go to the store, you buy the pie.

3) You approach the pie table. "That does smell delightful," you tell yourself. You see the blueberry pie. But wait—instead of automatically popping it into your cart, you decide to consider the facts and what your options are. You read the label and find the pie is high in saturated fat and sugar and has a number of chemical additives. It even has trans fat. And what are those artificial sweeteners doing in there along with the sugar? You decide you can make the pie yourself with less fat, less sugar, and no chemical additives. Maybe a friend or family member will make it with you. Maybe you'll take a stab at making it yourself and then freeze a portion of it if there's no one else around to eat it. Or maybe you'll make a healthy homemade blueberry cobbler instead. Or you'll look for a healthier frozen version of the pie.

Or you'll skip the pie idea altogether, buy some blueberries to eat, and save the rest of the money for something else...like gasoline.

Interesting, no? Outcome 1 depicts a complete lack of any type of willpower; outcome 2, misdirected use of willpower. Option 3, however, let's you look outside the pie box, literally, and make healthier choices. *That's* true willpower. This is not to say that an occasional junkfood indulgence is off limits. By no means. It's simply the frequency of such indulgences that's key. Practicing moderation — or better yet, *minimization* — should be your goal. When you find yourself craving a certain food, search out the healthiest version of it that tastes good. Or consider creating it yourself, if that's feasible. You'll be doing your body a favor while at the same time eliminating post-indulgence regrets.

Seeing Beyond The Obstacles

Employing willpower effectively does take some time and effort, but who better to invest in than yourself? And it really does get easier with time. You become savvy, informed, educated. You're able to read labels accurately in a snap, avoid questionable chemical ingredients, and recognize clever advertising tactics. You're in control from a lot of different standpoints and it feels good. And it's not difficult to achieve. You just have to want it—and not fall victim to the following two common misconceptions that can get in your way:

Misconception #1: "I have no willpower."

I hear this a lot. But it's just not true. You *do* have willpower. We all do. Willpower is in your back pocket 24/7/365. You can pull it out and use it anytime you feel like it. It's like a muscle; the more you use it, the stronger it becomes—and the easier it is to get things done with it. The important thing is knowing how to channel it productively with regard to food.

I once heard a doctor tell a woman who had serious clinical depression that whenever she felt her worst she should focus her energy on being productive at something positive. That way, he explained, things would actually *be* better when she felt better, and her life as a whole would start looking up. Best advice I've ever heard. Good advice to take when you're heading for that bucket of full-fat ice cream in the freezer with intent to devour it because you just lost your job or your partner left you. Why make things worse for yourself? Why set yourself back? It's far better to take hold of your willpower and put your determination in overdrive in a truly productive way, such as by improving your skills and looking for an even better job if you lost yours. That's the goal in the long run anyway, isn't it?

If you just have to have that ice cream, try not to binge. Consider keeping a low-fat version or some other

icy treat on hand for life's tougher days. Frozen bananas and other nutrient-packed whole frozen fruits are
good alternatives. Or find some other good-tasting
binge-friendly foods to keep on hand. In any case, try to
remember to put some thought into what you are putting
into your body, especially when you're under stress.
True, you rarely if ever see an actress in a movie reach
for a fresh, crisp apple or a crunchy carrot after she's
found out that her lover is cheating. But it might not be
a bad idea.

Interestingly, women tend to be emotional eaters.
Men just eat when they're hungry. When men are down,
they often lose their appetites and avoid food. That's
not good either. It can actually lead to weight gain later,
because the body readjusts itself to run on less food.

Misconception #2: "I can't cook."

This is another comment I hear a lot. My response:
learn how. Preparing food is a basic life essential. It's

part of self care. I'm not saying you have to become a master chef. Just learn how to prepare basic, healthy foods. Take a class, watch a health-related food show on TV, or read a book on preparing nutritious meals. Invest in yourself. It's not only empowering, it can also be a lot of fun. Just remember to stay focused on what's healthy (read: use willpower).

Be Strategic

Once you become educated about the potential benefits and deficits associated with different foods and beverages, choosing what to eat or drink will become second nature. Still feel like you need a leg up? Here are some tactics you can use to make it even easier:

- Try not to shop when you're hungry.
- Go on a shopping "field trip" to research different foods, or research them online.

- Shop for and make foods with your kids, your partner, or a friend.
- Never go to a party hungry.
- Bring healthy foods and snacks to conventions and events.
- Avoid drinking alcohol daily or in large quantities.
- If food is your sole source of pleasure, learn how to eat healthy *and* find an optional source of pleasure.
- Eat healthy, filling breakfasts and bring nutritious, tasty snacks to work. Then those donuts and bagels at the office won't look quite as inviting. You might just start a trend.
- Always keep your focus on a leaner, healthier, happier you.

Keep At It

Nothing good comes easy. But something good can become easy, including eating for life and health. And no, the foods don't all have to taste like cardboard or dog food. In fact, you may find that most of them taste better than the foods you eat now. Remember to practice "mind over flavor" when trying new things. I always say don't knock it until you try it—at least twice (unless, of course, you have a reaction to something). If you don't like a food raw or when it's cooked a certain way, try preparing it differently or even with different ingredients. Don't forget to think outside the box. All in all, most people end up finding a lot of healthy new foods to enjoy.

Where there's willpower, there's a way.

Chapter 4
Learning About Nutrition: A Benefit With Benefits

Having a solid understanding of nutrition is second only to truly caring about yourself in your quest for effective weight loss and management. Like working with a computer program in which you need to know the codes in order to run it effectively, you need to know your body's codes in terms of foods and nutrients. It's not only essential, but worth the effort.

And while it may seem challenging and confusing, it's really not as bad as it seems. It can even make for some pretty interesting conversation. Here are some important basic tips to get you started:

- The recommended total daily fiber intake for healthy adults up to age 50 is 25 grams for women and 38 grams for men (about 14 grams per thousand calories ingested). For healthy adults over 50 the daily amount is 21 grams for women and 30 grams for men.

- Foods high in fiber include pears, raspberries, popcorn, pistachios, whole grains, berries, oat bran, lentils, peas, and beans.

- The iron found in iron skillets can be absorbed by the body through foods. Women lose iron; men store it. Too much can make you sick. Cooking beef liver in an iron pan is a double-whammy dose.

- According to the CDC, iron deficiency is the most common nutritional deficiency in the United States.

- According to the National Institutes of Health, vitamin B_{12} deficiency affects between 1.5% and 15% of the public, afflicting mainly those who are elderly, alcoholic, have digestive disorders such as Crohn's disease or celiac disease, or are vegetarians or vegans. **Note: A deficiency of this vitamin can cause *irreversible* nerve damage.**

- Mango skins and cashew shells contain urushiol, the same toxic substance common to poison ivy, oak, and sumac. (Ever wonder why you never see cashews for sale in the shell?)

- Conventional bagels are *very* high in carbs. Especially important info to know if you're diabetic or pre-diabetic.

- Men get osteoporosis too.

- Men and women have different nutrient needs.

- Our nutrient needs change throughout our lives.

- Leaving fish, meat, or poultry out on the counter to defrost, or defrosting it in warm or hot water, can cause the bacteria that develop on it to create toxins that can be deadly when eaten. **You can't cook the toxins out.**

- Sometimes foods are treated with ethylene gas to hasten ripening. Foods that may be gassed include tomatoes, bananas, pears, mangoes, and lemons.

- Many people are deficient in both calcium and vitamin D.

- Champagne gets you drunk faster than most other alcoholic beverages due to the bubbles in it.

- Some chewing gums contain up to seven different sugar substitutes.

- Sugar alcohols such as isomalt, sorbitol, xylitol, and others ending in "itol" can cause gastric upset including gas, cramps, and diarrhea when eaten in large quantities (30-40 sugarless mints). They're often found in combination with each other in gums and mints. Some people are more sensitive to their effects than others.

Do A Little Research

Since eating is something you do on a regular basis, learning about *what* you're eating is nothing short of a really good idea. Besides, taking the time to learn about the nutritional value of foods and beverages pays off with big dividends. Not only does it allow you to avoid chemical additives—particularly the questionable ones—that your body has to filter out, but it also enables you to more readily make healthier choices that taste good. An easy way to begin: start a small notebook, virtual or otherwise, that you can take with you, and make notes about particular foods until you become more familiar with what they offer nutritionally. And check up on them regularly—ingredients often change.

Learn How To Read Labels

Learning how to read nutrition labels isn't that tricky once you get the hang of it. Mainly it's important not to be fooled by simply looking at the amount of fat, carbs, sugar, sodium, and other nutritional components listed. Look at the serving size and servings per container (see Figure 1 on the next page) and multiply as needed to get the calories, grams, or other units for the *actual* amounts you'll consume. Note that the serving size listed is one cup, and that the number of servings per container is *two*. So if you eat the entire container, you are actually consuming 520 calories worth (260 calories per cup x two servings). You'll also be getting 26 total grams of fat, 10 grams of saturated fat, and 4 grams of trans fat.

Nutrition Facts

Serving Size 1 cup (228g)
Servings Per Container 2

Amount Per Serving

Calories 260   **Calories from Fat** 120

	% Daily Value*
Total Fat 13g	**20%**
Saturated Fat 5g	**25%**
Trans Fat 2g	
Cholesterol 30mg	**10%**
Sodium 660mg	**28%**
Total Carbohydrate 31g	**10%**
Dietary Fiber 0g	**0%**
Sugars 5g	
Protein 5g	

Vitamin A 4%	•	Vitamin C 2%
Calcium 15%	•	Iron 4%

* Percent Daily Values are based on a 2,000-calorie diet. Your Daily Values may be higher or lower depending on your calorie needs:

Calories:	2,000	2,500
Total Fat	Less than 65g	80g
Sat Fat	Less than20g	25g
Cholesterol	Less than300mg	300mg
Sodium	Less than2.400mg	2,400mg
Total Carbohydrate	300g	375g
Dietary Fiber	25g	30g

Calories per gram:
Fat 9   •   Carbohydrate 4   •   Protein 4

Figure 1. Sample Nutrition Facts Label

Listen To Your Body

Here are some things your body wants you to know:

1. I like fiber. It keeps me running at my best.
2. I prefer natural foods.
3. I prefer fresh food.
4. I prefer whole food, not processed food.
5. I don't really like alcohol. I can tolerate a little now and then. It's a highly refined carbohydrate and it contains toxins that can really affect me. My liver helps me to metabolize fat, and when it's not functioning at its prime, well, you do the math. Besides, alcohol really does a number on the nutrients in me and there's no confirmed scientific proof that it benefits us.
6. You're not too sure about chemical additives. Neither am I. Let's err on the side of caution.
7. I really like it when you get to sleep by 10:30 p.m. It helps me stay slim.
8. I don't like trans fat. At all.

9. I like to be hydrated. My favorite beverage is good old-fashioned plain water.

10. The nutrients in me work together, in synergy. Please don't give me an abundance of only one unless our doctor says you have to. By the way, if you put healthy foods in me and generally avoid things that are unhealthy, we may not need any additional nutrients at all.

Keep It Real

Whenever possible, opt for whole, natural foods. Don't let diet sodas, highly refined foods, and foods with fillers, additives, and artificial sweeteners take the place of fruits, vegetables, grains, quality drinking water, and other healthy choices. Consider buying and eating organic for those foods that are known to be higher in pesticide residues (visit EWG.org for a current listing) or are known to be treated with other types of chemicals.

Make A Plan

Keep in mind that every time you open your mouth and put food in it it's either trick or treat for your body— and taste buds can be easily duped. To avoid the trap of being lured into eating large quantities of unhealthy foods that taste good, decide on tasty, healthy staple foods that you can eat for breakfast, lunch, dinner, and snacks and keep them on hand. For example, cooked oat bran with fruit is an excellent choice for breakfast or any other time of day, given that you aren't on any medications that restrict eating it. (Don't knock it 'til you've tried it.) It takes less than three minutes to prepare, is high in fiber and nutrients, and tastes great. Stock up on high-fiber, lower-sodium corn chips, low-fat cheese, and other foods that are quick and easy. And try your best to hit the Five Fruits & Vegetables A Day recommendation set by the USDA. Learning what your options are for commonly consumed food will help a lot. The following chart provides an overview.

Some potential options for healthier eating

Trade these:	For these:
Conventional pasta	whole grain or 50/50 (half regular, half whole grain) pasta; rice pasta
Cream sauce	tomato sauce or other vegetable-based sauce or sauce made with milk, low-fat Greek yogurt, low-fat sour cream, or a combination of these
Full-fat sour cream	low-fat or nonfat plain Greek yogurt
Butter	whipped light butter, olive oil spread (use sparingly)
Whole milk	1% milk
Cream, half & half	2% milk

Ice cream	low-fat versions; whole frozen bananas, grapes strawberries, or other fruit
Cream cheese	neufchatel cheese; reduced-fat cream cheese
Potato chips	air-popped popcorn with a bit of olive oil and a dash of Realsalt® (optional)
Baked goods	lower-sugar, lower-fat cakes, cookies, and other baked goods with fiber
White bread (low fiber)	whole grain or 50/50 (half regular, half whole grain), whole grain wraps & crackers
Jelly & Jam	all-fruit jelly, jam, preserves
Salad dressing	homemade salad dressing*

Lunch meat	sliced turkey or chicken; peanut butter/nut butter and all-fruit jam
Ground beef	ground turkey
Pork roast/ribs	pork tenderloin
Poultry, skin on	poultry, skin off (chicken, turkey, etc.)
Fried meats, poultry, & seafood	roasted, broiled, or grilled meats, poultry, & seafood (not overcooked)
Fried eggs	poached, boiled, or scrambled eggs (not overcooked)
Fried vegetables	steamed vegetables
French fries, potato skins, loaded potatoes	baked potatoes

Fettuccine Alfredo	spaghetti with tomato sauce
Traditional lasagna	vegetable lasagna; low-fat cheese lasagna
Meat	beans, grains, low-fat cheese
Tacos, burritos	lower-fat chicken tacos or burritos, bean burritos, vegetable fajitas (use sour cream and guacamole sparingly; consider low-fat versions)

* For a delicious homemade salad dressing try this recipe: 1 cup water, ¼ cup olive oil, 2 tablespoons apple cider vinegar, spices to your liking. Another option is to add a tomato (and/or any other salad vegetables) and

blend the mixture. Basically, blend your entire salad and pour it on your salad. Frontier Natural Products also sells Simply Organic sauce packets for salads, meat marinades, and more. Visit FrontierCoop.com. For more healthy recipes visit FoodSmart.org.

You are what you eat. Be amazing.

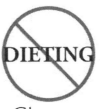

Chapter 5

Avoiding The Diet Trap:
How To Eat Right For Life

D iets don't work. Not as a lifelong solution to poor eating habits, anyway. Though I have seen people learn how to eat better as a result of going on a diet. The problem is they don't usually stick with it. Most people go from one diet to another, eventually giving up on dieting altogether and ending up weighing more than they did in the first place. Part of this is due to the fact that food restriction becomes a focus rather than the selection and consumption of healthy foods—that is, foods that are low in fat, sugar, sodium, and chemical additives and high in fiber and nutrients. And restriction is much easier to give up on than healthy eating options are.

Ironically, diet "shopping," or going from one diet to another, is actually most people's attempt to find a system of eating that allows them to lose weight, maintain a somewhat steady weight, or both. In other words, they're searching for those healthy eating options. They just don't realize it. They're caught in the diet trap. The good news is there's a way out: cut to the chase and learn how to eat right.

Synergy: The Real Weight-Loss Secret

We constantly hear about tips and tricks and secrets for weight loss. But in actuality the only truly effective method for achieving healthy weight loss and weight maintenance requires more than just changing what we eat. It also requires appropriate moderate exercise, proper hydration, relaxation, and sufficient sleep. In other words, it requires synergy.

Sleep, in particular, is an important yet often overlooked aspect of weight control. Obtaining it from the hours of approximately 10:30 p.m. to 6:30 a.m. helps our bodies do a lot of work to boost our immune systems and keep all of our other systems and hormones in check—including those that help us get and stay slim.

A Change Of Heart—And Heart Health

Seeking quick-fix weight loss solely for aesthetic reasons may provide the benefit of looking better, but it doesn't directly address any health issues. The fact is, being overweight or obese is hard on your heart. It's hard on your whole body. So if your main concern is how you look, try considering the health benefits of achieving and maintaining a healthy weight through good nutrition and beneficial lifestyle changes as opposed to dieting. The additional considerations can steer you toward long-term weight control. You're likely to not only look better, but also feel better and live longer.

Weight-Loss & Weight-Control Programs

The majority of weight-loss and weight-control programs are diets with some type of guidance thrown in, whether it be in the form of lists of foods you should and shouldn't eat, packaged meals, various recipes, or some combination of these. There are both pros and cons to such programs. For example, while those that include frozen packaged meals provide structure, convenience, and an easy way out for those who can't cook, they also create reliance on others, leave little if any control over the use of chemical additives in the foods being eaten, are often high in sodium, may not meet daily nutritional requirements, and can be inconvenient to store at work. They can also be expensive. Learning how to read labels and cook even the most basic of healthy foods puts *you* in the driver's seat. For life.

Adaptive Thermogenesis: Nature's Way of Saying "You Can't Trick Mother Nature"

Ever been on a diet where you lost about ten pounds the first week, seven or so the second week, about three or four the third week, and little or nothing the fourth week? It's mother nature's ingenious way of telling you that your body's basically in the equivalent state of being stranded on a mountaintop without food. The body naturally goes into emergency mode, rightfully protecting its resources. It begins to run on fuel reserve, holding onto the assets it has and latching on even tighter to any new ones it can get its cells on. It's called adaptive thermogenesis. Crash diets, fasting, and extreme food restrictions can throw the body into this state-of-emergency status even faster than conventional dieting from a number of different physical and mental standpoints, making them invitations for disaster in the same vein as constantly overeating and eating sodium-, sugar-, and fat-laden foods.

The Facts About Fasting

Highly restrictive sustained fasting is a rather scary concept. It can actually be dangerous, especially for those who are hypoglycemic or have thyroid problems or other medical conditions. This includes diabetics—and the thousands of people who are pre-diabetic and don't know it. Over the years I've seen countless people pass out and worse due to fasting. This includes people on fruit and vegetable juice fasts and spirulina fasts. The body is designed to run on healthy, nutritious, well-balanced food. If you've been eating less-than-healthy food, just switch over to the good stuff. That's all it takes. Your body will know the difference and make any necessary adjustments for the better. It's a really intelligent machine. There's no need to shock your system by first depriving it of food and then changing everything it's used to, unless your doctor says you have no choice. And don't forget that depriving your body of food can actually make you gain weight—or even make you lose too much.

The "Water Weight" Myth

I often hear people remark that they lost between five and ten pounds their first week on a diet and that what they lost was "water weight." In actuality, water retention is most often due to excess sodium intake or serious medical conditions (though there are other possible factors to consider, including menstruation or pregnancy). Healthy bodies don't harbor a gallon or so of extra water. Yet the myth is so commonly held that I constantly hear people say they actually stopped drinking water and most other beverages during their first week or two of dieting. Yikes! Truly not a good idea. Ironically, by drinking *more* water many people actually report *increased* weight loss. This is likely due to swapping water for calorie-laden drinks, feeling fuller from water consumption and eating less as a result, or both.

Weight Loss = Fat Loss + Muscle Loss

Another reason why dieting—particularly extreme dieting—isn't beneficial is the fact that when we loss fat we also lose muscle. For maximum effectiveness and ease on the body, weight loss should generally be a slow process (a pound or so a week) until the desired weight is reached, unless medical problems overseen by a certified doctor or specialist dictate otherwise. Appropriate moderate exercise should also be a part of the mix in order to maintain muscle tone. (For more information on exercise and weight, see chapter 8.)

The bottom line: the time, money, and energy spent going on diets is more effectively spent learning how to eat right for life.

Synergize!

Chapter 6
Shopping Effectively:
Ten Tips To Beat The System

In addition to the standard recommendation that you should never shop while you're hungry, here are ten other strategic tips to help you achieve effective shopping for healthy eating:

1) Read labels regularly. Ingredients change. This is due to a number of reasons, including cost increases, supply changes, and supplier issues.

2) Find out which foods are best bought organic (for info about pesticide residues visit EWG.org and the USDA's Pesticide Data Program).

3) Carefully read labels that say "lite," "light," "50% less fat," et cetera, or contain words such as "healthy" or "healthful." Be particularly cautious of low-calorie foods that are high in sugar.

4) Don't fall for "coupon allure." If something's a good deal, but it isn't good for you, it really isn't a good deal after all.

5) Compare prices. Note that in some cases the large economy sizes actually cost more than the smaller ones ounce for ounce.

6) Don't be sold by advertising and marketing "calls to action." Some examples: "buy some today," "try it," "get some now."

7) Learn which foods are generally high in sodium, fat, and sugar. Also learn which foods are generally low in sodium, fat, and sugar.

8) Make and take with you a menu list as well as a list of "swap out" foods that you can use in place of foods that are high in sodium, fat, and sugar.

9) Buy foods that contain "good" fats that are beneficial for your body. Use healthy oils to cook with. Extra virgin olive oil that is organic and first cold pressed is one of the best, particularly for adding to pasta dishes, salads, and air-popped popcorn.

10) Focus on fruit, vegetables, beans, legumes, and whole grains, and, unless you're a vegetarian or vegan, seafood and lean meats.

~~~

Avoid the Marketing Trap

When you shop, it's important to remember that stores are set up to make money. In the literal sense. Food product companies actually pay fees, often in the thousands, to display their products on end caps and in other prime locations. No, I'm not kidding. The goal is to get your attention; in other words, to get you to buy whatever it is they're selling. And what better way to do that than to play on your desire for foods that you think taste good, even if those foods are high in sodium, sugar, and unhealthy fats and contain a lot of chemical additives? (If you really want to be enlightened, just take a peek from a kid's eye level in a store.) Expend the time and effort to really think about what you're considering buying before you buy it. And remember not to fall for those "call to action" phrases, including "Buy some today," "Make it tonight," "Try it now," and others. See past the gimmicks and you'll be able to easily avoid being caught in the marketing trap.

Expand Your Portions Sizes, Not Your Waist

Let's face it—most portion sizes are pretty much, well, a joke. A one-inch square of cheese. Three quarters of a cup of cereal. A tablespoon of salad dressing. Really? That's not exercising willpower. That's torture. But what if the cheese were 75% reduced fat and still tasted delicious or the cereal were high in fiber and low in sugar and still tasted good? (See chapter 7 for suggestions on particular foods and brands.) We could increase the amount we eat, feel fuller, and not want to eat again ten minutes later.

The Truth About Organics

"Organic foods are too expensive."

If I had a dime for every time I've heard that. The truth is organic foods are often *less* expensive than conventional ones. Where you buy them is one major consideration; comparing prices is another. Knowing which foods to consider buying organic is yet another (visit

EWG.org for a list of foods that are higher in pesticide residues). Stocking up on storable organics when they're on sale is a great way to cut the cost even further. In addition, the major food warehouses now offer bulk organics of everything from meat and dairy products to fruit and vegetables. On top of all of this, many grocery store chains have regular weekly or bi-weekly sales on their organic produce and foods. And last but not least, don't forget about coupons.

Then there's the healthcare fees aspect. When you consider the cost to treat diseases likely brought on at least in part by chemicals, including those found in foods, organics suddenly become a bargain. Just check the cost to *attempt* to cure colon cancer alone these days. Not to mention that growing organics is healthier for the earth too.

When you further consider that most of us eat far more than we should at every sitting and much goes to waste, cutting back makes a lot of sense—and the cost of more expensive food (including some organics) levels out. Eating a smaller portion of food = less waste and less waist. And less money. Another win-win-win.

Education = power. Remember, you're in control.

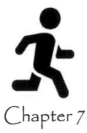

Chapter 7
Social & On-The-Go Eating: Strategies For Managing Meals

You're at a party and nearly everything is loaded with fat, sodium, and sugar. You're at a convention and the "lunch box" is more like a junk box. You're in a restaurant and most of the foods on the menu are fried. Sound all too familiar? Whether you're on a date at the fanciest restaurant in town or forced to make a choice out of an office building vending machine, knowing the nutritional value of foods comes in handy.

It's your number one tactic against weight gain *and* your number one tactic for weight loss.

Fortunately most packaged foods come with a cheat sheet: the nutrition label. And while you can't usually see the nutrition label on a bag of food hanging in a vending machine, choosing the whole grain chips over the candy bar is likely your best bet. But not necessarily. It depends on the overall ingredients each food contains and its fat, sodium, sugar, and fiber content, among other things. So reading labels whenever you have the chance is valuable, whether it be while you're shopping in the grocery store or browsing the internet for product information. With time you can become pretty much an expert at picking out the healthier stuff.

By the way, reading the *entire* label on packages, not just the nutritional information, is really important. Case in point: once while traveling I purchased a package of frozen, wild-caught, skinless salmon with no added preservatives or other chemicals — just the way I like it.

But I later realized that the bottom of the package read "Product of China." After a few phone calls I was informed that while the salmon was actually caught in the northwest, it had spent up to two months in China for processing before being returned to the United States. Uncomfortable with the idea that my fish had been vacationing in another country for up to eight weeks, I returned it to the store. My advice: look for the fine print. And the wandering print.

All in all, the labels for some foods will shock you; others will pleasantly surprise you. Still others will leave you a bit confused. Take for example a gum that's currently being distributed nationally. It has *seven* different sugar substitutes in it, including neotame (sister to aspartame, a.k.a. NutraSweet®), which is 7,000 to 13,000 times sweeter than sugar all by itself. Makes you wonder why there are six other sweeteners in the product.

So what about cases where there's no nutritional information on a package (such as often occurs in bakeries) or only the ingredients are listed and nothing else? If there's no information at all, you have three options: 1) ask the food manufacturer; 2) use sparingly; or 3) avoid. If there are only ingredients listed, they are generally shown in order of decreasing quantity in the product. For example, if a product's first ingredient is sugar, it likely contains more sugar than anything else in its ingredient list.

The good news is that while social and on-the-go eating both present their share of nutritional dilemmas, none of them are unsolvable. All it takes is some knowledge and preparation and a good game plan. Listed here are proven effective strategies to help you stay on track with both your weight-loss and weight-maintenance goals in different situations:

Snacks

Keeping healthy, low-fat snacks on hand is one of the most important moves you can make to take control of your weight. Make a snack pack—a small bag or other container that fits in your purse or briefcase—and refill it as needed. It's that simple. And it comes with the added bonus that you usually save money buying snack foods in quantity versus buying them on the run. Look for foods that are low in fat, sugar, and sodium, and high in fiber and nutrients. Alternate your daily snack selections to avoid flavor boredom.

◊ Low fat = 3 grams or less of fat per serving.

◊ A good source of fiber = 2.5 to 4.75 grams per serving; an excellent source of fiber = 5 grams per serving.

◊ Low sodium = 140 milligrams or less per serving.

◊ Keep added sugars at 5 milligrams or less per serving.

Some good potential snack pack options:

- Fresh nuts (particularly walnuts, which are rich in omega-3 fatty acids)

- popchips®
- Shelton's® Turkey Jerky
- Puffins® Original cereal
- Air-popped popcorn with a little olive oil and a dash of Redmond Real Salt®
- Organic apples
- Newman's Own® Organics Spelt Pretzels
- Michael Season's Popped Black Bean Crisps
- Homemade fruit and nut mixtures
- Cascadian Farms® cereals
- Beanitos® Black Bean Chips
- Way Better Snacks® Black Bean Tortilla Chips
- Mediterranean Snacks® Baked Lentil Chips
- Mary's Gone Crackers® Crackers

- Eden® Organic Seeds & Dried Fruits
- The Buffalo Guys™ Buffalo Jerky
- Cabot™ 50% and 75% Reduced Fat Cheeses

On-The-Run & Restaurant Drinks

Since beverages are often either high in sugar or filled with chemical additives, or both, it's best to opt for clean, good quality water whenever possible. A bottle of sweetened beverage that lists 30 grams of sugar on the label may actually contain 75 grams of sugar if the serving size states 2.5 servings. And indulging in that extra-large cup that the waitress just keeps filling up for you could cause you to top out at over 100 grams of sugar just from your drink alone.

Then there's coffee. Some designer coffee drinks have as much as ten grams of fat and about one fourth of your total daily calorie needs. Have two of them in the same day and you've consumed *half* of your recommended calories for the day. This can make it easy to pack in extra calories—and pack on extra pounds. The best bet if you want coffee: stick with good old-fashioned plain versions most of the time and indulge in the designer types once in a while. Asking for lower-fat milk and less flavoring syrup and sugar can help too. Also note that decaf coffee can actually contain *more* caffeine than regular coffee. Only caffeine-free coffees are truly caffeine free (or close to it).

Long, Busy Work Days

While you may want to indulge in a donut at the office now and then, making it a daily habit can be defeating to your weight-loss and weight-maintenance efforts. You can beat the system by searching out healthier alternatives to eat both before and during work. Reusable bags provide a handy way to transport dry and non-perishable foods and snacks, while small ice-pack totes designed specifically to keep cold foods cold are useful for transporting perishables. Both should be sanitized regularly. When possible, storing healthy snacks at work can also be beneficial.

Business Lunches

Choose light, healthy foods. A lightly grilled chicken breast or wild-caught fish with brown or wild rice and steamed vegetables (and no salty or fatty sauces) is a good example. Check the menu for "light" portions or ask if a smaller size is available. Don't forget to consider ordering appetizers if the standard portions are too large. Water with lemon is an excellent drink choice.

Conventions & Events

If you're attending a convention or event, ask about your lunch and snack options beforehand and choose accordingly, or bring your own. If you're exhibiting or presenting it's often best to make and take your own food. In either case, bring your own healthy snacks and water as a backup.

Road Trips

Consider the length of the road trip and where you're going. Realize that if you live in the city and have access to an abundance of stores and all the variety one could want, but are headed for the country, the food choices are likely to be more limited. Additionally, rest stops, travel plazas, and gas stations do not always provide the healthiest food and beverage options. Plan ahead. And always bring and drink sufficient water to fend off dehydration.

Parties

A few different strategies can work well for parties: eat light beforehand and snack while there; eat a complete meal before you go and snack little, if at all, while there; or don't eat before you go and make sensible choices and limit your overall consumption while there. Note that if you're already full of healthy, low-fat foods, you'll be less likely to attack the dessert table.

Beware of high-fat dips served with innocent-looking vegetables. It's easy to eat three days' worth of sat fat while thinking you're eating healthy. Ask for seltzer water with lemon, or fruit juice cut with seltzer water, instead of sugar-filled beverages. Keep alcohol consumption to a minimum. Take small samples of foods and decide on your favorites rather than taking large portions and feeling obligated to eat them. Avoid eating just because others are.

Eating At Restaurants

Generally speaking, when you're planning to eat at a restaurant:

- Prepare to eat a bigger overall meal and eat light in the hours beforehand.

- Keep portion sizes in mind.

- Avoid fried foods.

- Don't pig out on bread.

- Drink water or seltzer water, with or without lemon, rather than sugar-filled beverages.

- Always keep in mind that alcoholic beverages are calorie heavy.

- Avoid heavy cream sauces and gravies.

- Ask for salad dressings, sauces, and gravies on the side and use sparingly, particularly if cream-based.

- Choose baked foods over fried.

- Design your own dish or meal.

- Don't be afraid to order a la carte or build an a la carte meal.

- Use the Quota System (see chapter 2).

- Choose steamed vegetables.

- Choose baked potatoes in place of fries, loaded potatoes, and stuffed potato skins.

- Share a dessert—or skip it.

- Order a light portion (especially if you're going to the movies afterwards and plan to snack there).

- Select broiled or baked meat, fish, and poultry in place of fried.

- Consider your frequency of eating out and how it's affecting your weight.

- Check what's on the menu at different restaurants, make comparisons, and choose smart.

Eating Dinner At Someone's House

Generally speaking, when you're planning to eat at someone else's house:

- As with eating at restaurants, prepare to eat a bigger overall meal and eat light beforehand.

- If possible, serve yourself rather than allowing others to serve you.

- As with eating at parties or restaurants, ask for either water or seltzer water with or without lemon instead of heavily sugared drinks and keep alcohol consumption to a minimum.

- Don't feel obligated to finish or use up foods. If necessary, offer to take some home.

In General

- Be aware that ingredients often differ depending on how they're dispensed. For example, movie theater soda often contains ingredients not found in store-bought soda, and restaurant spin-off foods found in the freezer sections of supermarkets often have different ingredients than those used in the actual restaurants.

- Be confident in your dietary choices.

- Ignore peer pressure. Don't feel obligated to eat what your friends are eating.

- Always graciously and confidently respond to any comments about your dining habits.

- Never engage in binge-purge activities, which are common among college students. They cause broken blood vessels in your face and eyes; damaged tooth enamel; esophagus problems, and other less-than-appealing aesthetic and health-related effects.

Knowledge + preparation = the solution.

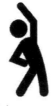

Chapter 8

The Exercise Connection:
Why Physical Activity
Is Essential

D ust off your treadmill. Oil that old exercise bike. Get out your walking shoes. Physical activity is a vital part of achieving and maintaining a healthy weight. It also keeps your heart healthy, your joints flexible, your muscles and bones strong, your cancer risk lower, your spirits up, and your brain alert. And it comes with an added bonus: it boosts your Basal

Metabolic Rate (BMR), which helps you burn more calories. You can't beat it. But that doesn't mean you should go grazing through the kitchen after a workout, or indulge in a high-fat, high-sugar dessert after dinner. What it does mean is that you'll be on your way to a slimmer, healthier you, particularly if you watch your food intake too.

Note that the exercise need not be strenuous or excessive. Walking your dog to the neighbor's mailbox doesn't count, however. Unless it's at least half an hour or so away.

So how much exercise do you actually need? Well, that depends on you—as an individual. It can vary dramatically from one person to another, though the general consensus is that between two and three hours of moderate-intensity aerobic activity; 75-90 minutes of vigorous-intensity aerobic activity; or an equivalent combination of the two each week should do the trick for maintaining weight. To lose weight you also need to cut back on calories. (That doesn't mean you need to *count* calories, but rather that you need to avoid or eat smaller portions of some foods you know are calorie dense.)

So how do you measure moderate activity? For starters, you can tell if it's moderate if you're able to talk, but not sing, while you're doing it. For example, you can talk while you walk briskly, but not while you jog. Jogging is more of a vigorous-intensity activity.

Moderate-intensity exercise includes:

- Brisk walking (approximately 3-4 mph)
- Biking (under 10 mph)
- Simple gardening
  (no excessive digging, raking, or weed pulling)
- Mowing using a push mower
  (self-propelled mowers don't count)
- Water aerobics

Vigorous-intensity exercise includes:

- Jogging

- Running

- Swimming laps

- Rollerblading or inline skating at a brisk pace

- Cross-country skiing

- Most competitive sports (football, basketball, or soccer)

- Jumping rope

Intensity varies on exercise machines according to settings, and you can work your way up.

The following table provided by the Centers for Disease Control shows the approximate amount of calories used in common physical activities at both moderate and vigorous intensity levels:

Moderate Physical Activity	Approximate Calories/Hr for a 154 lb Person[1]
Hiking	370
Light gardening/yard work	330
Dancing	330
Golf (walking and carrying clubs)	330
Bicycling (<10 mph)	290
Walking (3.5 mph)	280
Weight lifting (general light workout)	220
Stretching	180

Vigorous Physical Activity	Approximate Calories/Hr for a 154 lb Person[1]
Running/jogging (5 mph)	590
Bicycling (>10 mph)	590
Swimming (slow freestyle laps)	510
Aerobics	480
Walking (4.5 mph)	460
Heavy yard work (chopping wood)	440
Weight lifting (vigorous effort)	440
Basketball (vigorous)	440

Getting & Staying Motivated

For many people, losing or maintaining weight is enough of an incentive to start exercising. But there are also a lot of other benefits, including increased muscle tone, firmer skin, and better sleep, to name a few. The important thing is that you don't let getting a head cold, working late, watching a TV series, having friends visit, or anything else interrupt your regimen for too long. Why? Because it can be tempting to stop. Exercise is work, but it's *really valuable* work. Don't give up on it. The rewards are just too great. Exercise with a friend or a group if necessary, but also set up an exercise regimen of your own for days when you need or want to exercise alone. Consider light weights, a jump rope, and various exercise machines for in-home use. (You can strategically place your treadmill or exercise bike in front of the television so you won't miss that TV series.) Set up a calendar and mark off the days you exercise. That way you can see your accomplishments from more than one angle.

Send fat walking, literally.

Chapter 9
Media, Moms & Models:
Staying Realistic

S uper-skinny actresses. Anorexic models. Four-
year-olds on diets. It's the flipside of obesity—
and it's not pretty. The drive toward being thin
has caused a lot of people, mainly females, to fall victim
to placing aesthetics over health. The unrealistic expec-
tations associated with being ultra-thin are a setup for
disaster, leading to eating disorders and other physical

and emotional problems. Left unaddressed, they can set the stage for lifelong health issues that affect every area of a person's life.

Sadly, and ironically, eating disorders often get their roots at home, during childhood and adolescence. But then so does obesity. Kids whose moms and dads have eating disorders or are obese often face the same difficulties themselves. Fortunately there's a solution. Learning about food and nutrition and eating well-balanced, good-tasting meals and snacks are beneficial and effective ways to keep the scale balanced.

Media

Much of the media continually focuses on the weight status of celebrities from the moment they're born, holding them under a magnifying glass of scrutiny and slamming them for even the slightest weight changes all in the name of profit. The irony is that most of the writers who develop such stories eat poorly and are overweight or obese themselves. It's important, especially for children and teens, to realize that celebrities are real people; people who often have their own food issues and fight their own battles with weight problems.

Moms

Moms have much influence on the health and well-being of their children. For that matter, so do dads, though usually not to quite as great an extent. On one hand, well-meaning moms often "accidentally" push their daughters to maintain super-slim figures, usually with the mindset that by being thin they will have an easier time finding a marriage partner. On the other hand, mothers' preoccupation with their own weight often invisibly gives their daughters the message that being less than ultra skinny makes a woman a devastating failure. Most moms —and dads (and people in general)—don't realize the impact of making negative comments about weight to a child or teen. Taking your influence and using it to teach kids and teens about food and nutrition, including how to shop for healthy foods and cook, is a priceless, everlasting gift. It's the ultimate hand-me-down. And it's a lot more effective than the nagging and demeaning route.

Models

Imagine waking up, eating something, and throwing it up shortly thereafter. Further imagine that in the interim, before vomiting, you apply chemical-filled spray tan to your body, hemorrhoid cream under your eyes, and hairspray to your backside. No, you didn't read that wrong. Sounds wild? These aren't uncommon events in the lives of many models. And that's just a sample.

A little over a decade ago, I boarded a plane to go talk about nutrition on a television show. A nineteen-year-old female sat in the seat directly across from me. Her feet were black with dirt, her hair stiff and tangled. She smelled awful. Before takeoff she downed some type of food in a bag (without ever exposing it), then entered the lavatory, vomited fiercely, and returned to her seat. I must have looked appalled, because she stared directly at me and said, "I'm a model. This is what we do. It's not all as glamorous as it seems. It's a really hectic and demanding lifestyle."

It was a startling—and enlightening—moment. She was going through so much misery. For what? Like ballerinas who perform with incredible grace throughout their careers only to be severely crippled in their older years due to extensive damage to their feet, models who deprive their bodies of essential nutrition and other basic needs will pay far too heavy a price later on. That price will likely include osteoporosis and dentures, just for starters.

The point is, you don't need to look like a model. And your ideal weight isn't necessarily what's posted on a chart in your doctor's office. It may be a few pounds more, or a few pounds less. It's the weight at which you feel your best and are the healthiest, not the weight of the model on the commercial for diet pills who's never even taken one. You don't need to be stick thin. Neither do your kids.

Focus on healthy. The happy will follow.

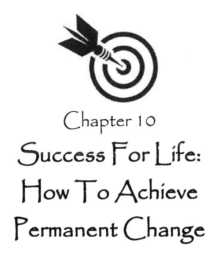

Chapter 10

Success For Life: How To Achieve Permanent Change

I t's all about dedication and determination. It's for those who want to win the war against overweight and obesity, not those who just think about it now and then. It's for those who make a plan—a life plan—and stick with it. It's for *you*. And it's achievable, without excessive exercise, constant food restrictions, or eating tasteless or bad-tasting foods.

One of the keys to being truly successful at losing and maintaining weight is not talking about it, but rather just *doing* it. Another is realizing that it isn't only about watching what you eat. It's about living healthy as a whole. This includes learning about food and making better, healthier choices. Most people find it leads them to actually eat more, and to enjoy a much broader variety of delicious, nutrient-packed food.

Define Your Personal Relationship With Food

Do you regularly wake up looking forward to eating a bowl of heavily sugared cereal, followed by a heavily sugared cup of coffee with cream? Do you daydream about eating a chocolate brownie covered with vanilla ice cream while you're working? If you do, it's likely that you view food solely as a source of pleasure, without regard to the actual effects it can have on your body. Learn to see food as a source of nutrition too, rather than only a taste quencher.

Get—and Stay—Educated About Nutrition

Learn about foods and how to read labels. You'll empower yourself to take control of your weight, your health, and your life. It's a freedom like few others.

Expand Your Food Horizons

Try new foods and new ways of making foods. Branch out! Consider taking a nutrition or cooking class and reading about foods and food preparation.

Follow Your Own Path

Never lose sight of the fact that what you think about yourself matters most. When it comes down to it, you're the only person you really need to impress. Take a vested interest in *you*. Every day offers new opportunities for self-care and self improvement. The investment you make in yourself is worth it. It's a journey that will lead you to conquer your weight—and who knows what else.

Ignore anyone who dismisses your efforts unless you're somehow becoming unhealthy. Be confident in knowing that you're making the best choices. And don't be afraid to tell people what you don't want to eat. If your friends constantly eat junk food and binge on buffets, decline gracefully or go along and eat right. Find new friends if you have to. It's okay to judge the situation and the actions of other people. As I once heard a famous life coach say, "You judge somebody every time you choose a toilet paper." So judge on—and move on if necessary.

Make Exercise A Habit

No matter whether you have a tight schedule, heavy responsibilities, or physical limitations, find a way to exercise. Make it a part of your routine. It simply offers too many benefits to skip doing. Avoid excuses. Stay focused on the fact that you are making yourself into a healthy, lean powerhouse.

The Big Thirty

The following is a life map of 30 tips that can effectively help you beat overweight and obesity permanently. Read and re-read it as necessary.

1.   Learn about and care for your body. The better you treat it, the likelier it'll be to return the favor.

2.   Find an interest. Take up a hobby. Or donate your time to a good cause. Find an outlet other than eating. Boredom can lead to overeating.

3.   Address any depression problems that may cause you to overeat.

4.   Remember that stress can disrupt the body's systems—and poor eating habits add fuel to the fire. Be aware of this vicious cycle, as it can readily lead to overeating.

5.   Find out if you have allergies or sensitivities to any foods and avoid those items.

6.   Use your willpower effectively (see chapter 3).

7.   Learn about foods and beverages. Keep a small journal or notebook, virtual or otherwise.

8.   Learn how to read labels.

9.   Learn how to cook.

10.   Don't be swayed by advertising and marketing of foods that are high in sodium, fat, sugar, or chemical additives.

11.   Realize your personal or emotional attachment to a particular food and work with it—or around it.

12.   Set a quota for junk food intake.

13.   Curtail or eliminate your alcohol and sugared drink consumption.

14.   Create healthy alternatives of your favorite junk foods.

15.   Practice mind over flavor. Take the time to really think about whether a food or beverage is good

for you or not before you indulge in it. Reading labels comes in handy here.

16.   Don't knock a food until you've tried it—at least twice (unless you have a reaction to it or another reason to avoid it). Consider trying it in a different form if you don't like it at first.

17.   Always look for the healthiest, or at least healthier, alternatives.

18.   Find a way to make healthy food taste good and still be healthy.

19.   Keep healthy snacks on hand, particularly when working and traveling.

20.   Vary the types of foods you eat to prevent dietary boredom.

21.   Eat a balanced diet. Be sure to add high-fiber foods like pears, raspberries, whole grains, and air-popped popcorn.

22. Eat at least five fruits and vegetables a day.

23. Limit eating purely for pleasure. Eat mainly to satisfy hunger, and fill that hunger with quality nutrition.

24. Use the Quota System (see chapter 2).

25. Add healthy exercise to your routine. Remember that some is better than none—and more is generally better than a little. Jumping jacks work virtually every part of your body and they don't require any exercise equipment. They're the perfect travel exercise.

26. Get to sleep by 10:30 p.m. and get at least seven to eight hours of sleep.

27. Drink a cup of water with a teaspoon of lemon juice in it at least once a day.

28. Always practice the Oxygen Mask Theory (see chapter 1).

29. Don't worry if you falter. Get back on track and keep going.

30. Make eating healthy a way of life, not just a passing whim.

Be focused. Have determination. Be healthy. It will lead to a different, better life. You *can* do it.

Index

Ordering Information

Copies of **Me, Myself & Food** are $12.95 plus shipping ($3.50 Media Mail; $5.50 Priority Mail). Florida residents please add 6% sales tax. Checks and money orders (U.S. funds only) accepted.

By Mail: Consumer Press
            Order Department
            13326 Southwest 28th Street
            Suite 102
            Fort Lauderdale, FL 33330-1102

Online: www.consumerpress.com

Credit: MasterCard and Visa Only
            800-266-5752

See more about this author at FoodSmart.org.